Six-Minute Social Skills - 1

Conversation Skills for Kids with Autism & Asperger's

Six-Minute Social Skills

Happy Frog Learning

About Happy Frog Learning

Happy Frog Learning creates high-quality resources for elementary and high school-aged children with autism and other social/language challenges.

We believe that all children can learn – as long as we provide a learning environment that suits their needs.

www.HappyFrogLearning.com

Table of Contents

Introduction: Six Minute Social Skills 1

    How to Coach a Six-Minute Session 2

Topic 1 Discover Shared Interests 7

    Background 7

    1.1 Interests I Share With My Mom 9

    1.2 Interests I Share With My Friends 11

    1.3 Talk About What We Are Interested In 13

    1.4 Talk About Shared Interests 15

    1.5 Ask a 'Favorite' Question 17

    1.6 Ask About Recent Activities 19

    1.7 Listen to Find Shared Interests 21

    1.8 Shared Interests Review 23

Topic 2 Decide What to Talk About 25

    Background 25

    2.1 Think About What I Know 28

    2.2 Choose a Shared Interest 30

    2.3 Ask About Something Recent 32

    2.4 Ask For New Information 34

    2.5 Remember Previous Conversations 36

    2.6 Listen for Clues 38

    2.7 Follow My Friend's Clues 40

    2.8 Check for Current Topic 42

    2.9 Choosing a Topic: Review 44

Topic 3 Show I Am Listening 46

    3.1 Add a Short Comment 48

    3.2 Match the Emotion 50

3.3 Vary What I Say 52

3.4 Use Eyes and Body 54

3.5 Let's Practice 56

3.6 Review 58

Topic 4 Ask a Follow-up Question 60

4.1 Ask a Follow-up Question 62

4.2 Make It Related 64

4.3 Ask for New Information 66

4.4 Keep to My Friend's Topic 68

4.5 Use Open Questions 70

4.6 Let's Practice Open Questions 72

4.7 Look When I Start Talking 74

4.8 Review 76

Topic 5 Add a Follow-up Comment 78

5.1 Add a Follow-up Comment 80

5.2 Make It Related 82

5.3 Give New Information 84

5.4 Use Variety 86

5.5 Use My Eyes & Body 88

5.6 Review 90

Topic 6 Make Conversation 92

6.1 Use Variety 94

6.2 Let's Practice 96

6.3 Two Turns Each 98

6.4 Three Turns Each 100

6.5 Four Turns Each 102

6.6 Review 104

Need More Resources? 107

Introduction: Six Minute Social Skills

Welcome to the *Six Minute Social Skills* series. This series is designed for busy parents and professionals who need easy-to-use and effective materials to work with learners who have Autism, Asperger's and similar social skill challenges.

This book, *Six Minute Social Skills: Conversation Expert* provides step-by-step activities that develop strong conversation skills. By following through the activities, your student will learn how to:

- Discover his friend's interests in order to be able to talk about them.
- Choose a topic of interest to his friend and avoid focusing on his own special interests.
- Show he is listening with appropriate body language and comments.
- Respond to a friend with appropriate follow-up questions and follow-up comments.
- Identify when a topic is in progress and not barge in.
- Participate in multi-turn conversations, remaining on-topic and showing interest in his friends.

These skills are developed incrementally, with lots of practice, allowing your learner to make meaningful progress week by week.

The book contains forty-three activity pages, organized into 6 key skill areas. Each set of activities is preceded by a parent/educator guide containing suggestions for alternate and extension activities.

Children with ASD need strong conversation skills. This workbook is the guide you need to ensure their success.

How to Coach a Six-Minute Session

We want you and your learner to have fun when you coach a six-minute session. So here are some suggestions.

1. Don't worry if you never write in the book!

Conversation is an oral skill. Filling in pages is NOT practicing conversation.

So use the workbook as you need. Use it as a guide for discussion, a guide for oral practice, as an actual worksheet... whatever helps your student learn something new.

2. Don't be afraid to repeat.

In the six-minute series, we have broken down conversation skills into tiny steps. But even so, your learner will not develop these skills instantly. Don't be afraid to repeat an activity until your learner develops confidence.

If you are concerned about boredom, mix your review in with new lessons. In any case, don't move too far ahead if your learner still needs help with earlier skills.

3. Make sure to reciprocate.

A great way to learn is to be the teacher. Once your learner shows progress at a skill, switch the tables so that **you** have to reply. Get your learner to tell you what's wrong with your response.

4. Have a consistent schedule.

Consistency is important if you want to reach a goal. Choose a regular schedule for your six-minute sessions. Get your learner's agreement and stick to it!

We also recommend having a consistent method for delivering each six-minute session. This allows you to move quickly and helps your learner stay focused. Here's a schedule we have found successful.

1. Review the last lesson

Briefly review the Key Idea and activity from the most recent worksheet. Allow the student to see the worksheet as you discuss it.

> *Let's get started. Here's what we did last time. Do you remember what the Key Idea was for that lesson?*
>
> *<wait for student response>*
>
> *Right. And what did this diagram show?*
>
> *<wait for student response>*
>
> *Awesome. Let's see what we do today.*

2. Introduce today's Key Idea

All lessons have a Key Idea. This is a simple concept that is useful for students to be aware of. Once you have introduced a Key Idea, you can reference it when needed during everyday life.

For example, once you have introduced the key idea of talking about shared interests, you can remind your learner when he or she talks only on his/her own interests.

During a lesson, use a 3-step process to introduce the Key Idea.

1. READ:

Get your learner to read the key idea, or read it for your student if reading is a challenge.

> *Here is today's key idea. Can you read it for me?*

2. PARAPHRASE:

After the student has read the key idea, briefly paraphrase it in a way that is useful for your student's comprehension level.

> *Good reading! So, I guess that is saying that we all have different interests but often we can find things that we are both interested in.*

3. CONNECT:

Talk with your learner about the key idea. Can they think of any examples in their life where the key idea is relevant?

3. Complete & review the activity sheet

You can fill in the activity page by writing or complete it orally. Either approach is effective.

Provide whatever support is needed to complete the activities. Keep in mind that your goal for every activity is for your learner to reach the point where they can demonstrate the skill independently.

Once the activity sheet is complete, review it together. If your student finds this difficult, you can provide a model. Describe or paraphrase what the student has written/said. Where possible, relate it back to the key idea. For example:

> *I see that you are interested in quite a few things. You like swimming, hiking, going to the toy store and playing Minecraft. Your mom likes some of these things, too. She likes swimming and hiking, but she doesn't like playing Minecraft.*
>
> *That's really interesting.*
>
> *I can see that you have several shared interests. You both like swimming and hiking.*

4. Extra practice (optional)

Your learner may need extra practice. Most worksheets have suggestions for how to extend the skill development.

5. Revisit the Key Idea

To finish up, draw your learner's attention back to the Key Idea. Ask them to tell you the key idea and then ask your student a question that relates the key idea to the activity sheet or to the student's life.

> *Nice job. Now let's look at the Key Idea again. What was our Key Idea?*
>
> *<wait for student response>*
>
> *Yes. You and your mom each have your own interests, but you share some interests. What shared interests do you and your mom have?*
>
> *<wait for student response>*
>
> *Fantastic! Yes, you and your mom both like hiking. That is a shared interest.*

6. Congratulate your learner & finish

You should provide encouraging feedback throughout the six-minute session. Make sure to also finish up on a positive note. Congratulate your student and identify something they did well during the session.

Have fun!

FREE DOWNLOAD

Download the Key Ideas Summary PDF at:

HappyFrogLearning.com/product/Conversation_Key_Ideas

Topic 1
Discover Shared Interests

Background

Our first topic is learning about shared interests.

It is important to know about shared interests because most conversations focus on topics that are interesting to both participants. Children with Autism often talk about their own special interests instead of shared interests and may not be aware that the other person is not interested.

In this chapter, we step the learner through the process of thinking about what interests they share with important people in their life. Your student will learn that shared interests will be different from person to person.

The student will also practice 3 strategies for identifying their friend's interests.

1. Asking a 'favorite' question
2. Asking a 'What did you do...' question
3. Listening to what their friend talks about

These strategies will help students learn more about their friends and have more topics to talk about.

Coaching Guide: Interests I Share With My Mom

Quick Reference:

» Introduce the 'Six Minute Social Skills' workbook

» Introduce the Key Idea: Read, paraphrase, connect

» Complete & review the worksheet

» Extra practice

» Revisit the Key Idea

» Congratulate your learner & finish

General Notes: The worksheet uses 'mom' as the comparison. Feel free to replace 'mom' with someone equally important in your learner's life.

Extra Practice: Choose another important person in your student's life. Get your student to describe that person's interests and to identify which interests your student shares with this individual.

Your goal is to get your learner thinking about shared interests without needing the visual support of the chart. If your student struggles, draw a chart for them to use on a blank piece of paper.

If your student continues to need visual support, redo the worksheet in your next session for additional practice. It is important that your student develop fluency in thinking about other people's interests.

After Session: In everyday life, encourage your learner to identify the interests they share with friends they encounter.

Your Notes/Extra Ideas:

1.1 Interests I Share With My Mom

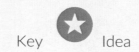

Key Idea

My mom and I each have our own interests.

Some of our interests are **shared interests**.

Fill in the chart:

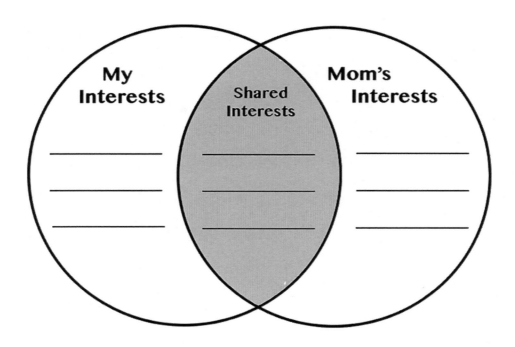

My mom and I share an interest in_____.

My mom likes _____, but I don't.

I like _____, but my mom doesn't.

Coaching Guide: Interests I Share With My Friends

Quick Reference:

> » Review the last worksheet
>
> » Introduce the Key Idea: Read, paraphrase, connect
>
> » Complete & review the worksheet
>
> » Extra practice
>
> » Revisit the Key Idea
>
> » Congratulate your learner & finish

General Notes: Draw attention to the shared interests to show how the interests your student shares with his first friend/family member are different from the interests your student shares with the second friend/family member.

Extra Practice: Choose an additional friend/family member for your student to practice without visual support.

After Session: Get your learner to think about interests they share with friends they encounter this week.

Your Notes/Extra Ideas:

1.2 Interests I Share With My Friends

My shared interests are different, depending on who I am thinking about.

Fill in the charts, one for each friend:

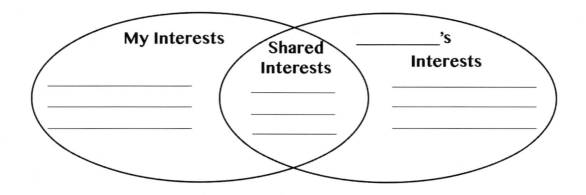

My friend _____ and I are both interested in _____.

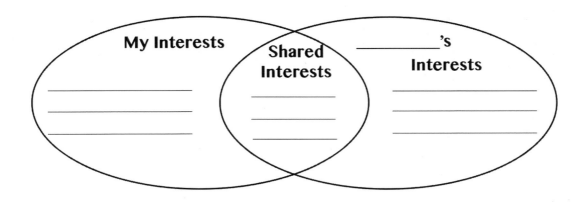

My friend _____ and I are both interested in _____.

Coaching Guide: Talk About What We Are Interested In

Quick Reference:

>> Review the last worksheet

>> Introduce the Key Idea: Read, paraphrase, connect

>> Complete & review the worksheet

>> Extra practice

>> Revisit the Key Idea

>> Congratulate your learner & finish

General Notes: Shared interests are excellent topics for conversation. This lesson introduces this important idea to your learner. The concept will be reinforced in later worksheets.

Extra Practice: Choose another friend and verbally complete the questions from the worksheet with reference to that friend. Continue if more practice is needed.

After Session: If your learner chooses to talk about her own special interests a lot, occasionally remind her to think about shared interests and choose a more appropriate topic to talk about.

Also, prime your learner before encounters with family members or friends. Ask your learner to identify a shared interest or two before they talk to their friend.

Your Notes/Extra Ideas:

1.3 Talk About What We Are Interested In

Everyone likes to talk about things they are interested in.

Likes

Video Games

Dogs

Skiing

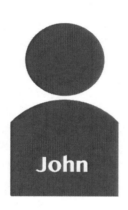

Does Not Like

Hiking

Snakes

Ice cream

Complete the sentences.

I think John likes to talk about _____ and _____ .

I think John does not like to talk about _____ .

When I talk to John, I could talk about _____ .

Coaching Guide: Talk About Shared Interests

Quick Reference:

> » Review the last worksheet

> » Introduce the Key Idea: Read, paraphrase, connect

> » Complete & review the worksheet

> » Extra practice

> » Revisit the Key Idea

> » Congratulate your learner & finish

General Notes: Today's message is very important for ASD learners as they tend to focus on their own special interests.

Extra Practice: Choose another friend and verbally complete the questions from the worksheet with reference to that friend. Your learner will first identify some shared interests and then choose two that they could talk about.

If your learner does not know what their friend is interested in, don't worry. This is typical for ASD kids. You will work on discovering a friend's interests in the next few worksheets

After Session: Be prepared for lots of gentle reminders about choosing a topic that both participants are interested in. Priming ahead of time is an excellent practice. Fade when your learner starts choosing appropriate topics independently.

Your Notes/Extra Ideas:

1.4 Talk About Shared Interests

When I talk, I should choose a topic my friend and I are both interested in.

Look back at worksheet 1.2 and answer the following questions.

Friend # 1

My friend's name is _____ .

When I talk to him/her, I can talk about _____ or _____.

My friend might get bored if I talk too much about _____ .

Friend # 2

My friend's name is _____ .

When I talk to him/her, I can talk about _____ or _____.

My friend might get bored if I talk too much about _____ .

Coaching Guide: Ask A 'Favorite' Question

Quick Reference:

>> Review the last worksheet

>> Introduce the Key Idea: Read, paraphrase, connect

>> Complete & review the worksheet

>> Extra practice

>> Revisit the Key Idea

>> Congratulate your learner & finish

General Notes: Often children with ASD do not pay attention to their friend's interests. So it can be difficult for them to choose an appropriate shared interest. The next three worksheets teach students simple strategies for discovering what their friends are interested in.

Extra Practice: Encourage your learner to practice this question with friends and family. If helpful, create a chart of your learner's friends and their interests. Your student can gradually fill in the chart as they talk to their friends and family and use the 'What is your favorite ____?' question.

Consider providing a reward for completing the whole chart.

After Session: Before and after encounters with friends and family, engage your learner in a discussion about what their friend/family member is interested in. Prompt or prime your learner to ask a 'favorite' question to learn more about their friend/family member.

Your Notes/Extra Ideas:

1.5 Ask a 'Favorite' Question

I can find out my friend's interests by asking,

"What is your favorite _____?"

Make up some sentences to find out a friend's interests:

What is your favorite _____*movie*_____ ?

What is your favorite _____ ?

What is your favorite _____ ?

What is your favorite _____ ?

Choose one of these questions and ask your coach or someone nearby.

Then fill in these sentences.

I talked to _____ .

His/her favorite _____ is _____ .

I know _____ is interested in _____ , so I can talk

to him/her about _____ .

Coaching Guide: Ask About Recent Activities

Quick Reference:

» Review the last worksheet

» Introduce the Key Idea: Read, paraphrase, connect

» Complete & review the worksheet

» Extra practice

» Revisit the Key Idea

» Congratulate your learner & finish

General Notes: It is important for learners to have a variety of strategies for learning about their friends. You do not want them to become rigid and always ask the same question.

Extra Practice: Encourage your learner to practice these questions with friends and family. If your learner is ready, expand their skillset to include questions about what friends are doing in the future. For example, "What are you doing this weekend?"

After Session: Ask your learner to practice these questions in their daily life and report back to you next session.

Your Notes/Extra Ideas:

1.6 Ask About Recent Activities

I can find out my friend's interests by asking,

"What did you do last _____?"

Make up some sentences to find out a friend's interests:

What did you do last ___ *weekend*_____ ?

What did you do _____ ?

What did you do _____ ?

What did you do_____ _____ ?

Choose one of those questions and ask your coach. Then fill in these sentences.

I talked to _____ .

Recently, he/she _____.

From this I know he/she is interested in _____ , so I can talk to him/her about _____ .

Coaching Guide: Listen To Find Shared Interests

Quick Reference:

> » Review the last worksheet
>
> » Introduce the Key Idea: Read, paraphrase, connect
>
> » Complete & review the worksheet
>
> » Extra practice
>
> » Revisit the Key Idea
>
> » Congratulate your learner & finish

General Notes: This worksheet may be difficult for a child who:

- Does not attend to their peer's conversation
- Does not participate in conversations
- Did not participate in a conversation recently

No problem! That's why you are doing this workbook.

If your child can't access information by recalling real-life conversations, you have several options.

Find a conversation to listen to... without invading anyone's privacy of course! Are there any other family members you can prompt to have a conversation? Other staff members? Peers? Can you prompt your learner to pay attention during family dinner to see what topics family members introduce?

If there are no real-life conversations around you, practice by using segments from a favorite movie or TV show.

If you have to use these alternate strategies, make sure you spend a few days on this worksheet and work with your child until they can report on a conversation they participated in with their peers.

Your ultimate goal is for your child to learn about what their peers are interested in by attending to the topics they introduce.

After Session: Get your student to report back next session about a shared interest they determined from listening.

Your Notes/Extra Ideas:

1.7 Listen to Find Shared Interests

I can find out my friend's interests by...

Listening to the topics he or she chooses to talk about.

Think back to a conversation that you were part of today. What topics did your friend introduce?

My friend _____ talked about _____ .

I can guess my friend is interested in _____.

My friend _____ talked about _____ .

I can guess my friend is interested in _____.

My friend _____ talked about _____ .

I can guess my friend is interested in _____.

Coaching Guide: Shared Interests Review

Quick Reference:

> » Review the last worksheet
>
> » Introduce the Key Idea: Read, paraphrase, connect
>
> » Complete & review the worksheet
>
> » Extra practice
>
> » Revisit the Key Idea
>
> » Congratulate your learner & finish

General Notes: Use today's time to review the three strategies your student has learned to find out a friend's interests.

- Ask 'favorite' questions
- Ask 'What did you do...?' questions
- Listen to the topics your friends talk about

Extra Practice: Ask about conversations your learner had during the week. What do they know about their friends' interests from those conversations?

After Session: After encounters with friends/family, ask your learner what topics they talked about and what they can guess about their friends' interests and likes.

Your Notes/Extra Ideas:

1.8 Shared Interests Review

I talk to my friends about things we are both interested in.

I know three ways to find out my friend's interests.

To find out my friend's interests I can:

1. _____

2. _____

3. _____

Topic 2
Decide What to Talk About

Background

In this section, students practice choosing appropriate topics.

Early lessons focus on using appropriate **topic-starter questions**. A topic-starter question can be used to start a conversation with a friend or begin a new topic during a conversation. Students use information about shared interests to ask appropriate topic-starter questions.

Students will learn that topic-starter questions:

- Should be about their friend's interests.
- Should be about recent events or activities.
- Should ask for new information

Students next learn how to follow clues from their friend to know what their friend wants to talk about.

Coaching Guide: Think About What I Know

Quick Reference:

» Review the last worksheet

» Introduce the Key Idea: Read, paraphrase, connect

» Complete & review the worksheet

» Extra practice

» Revisit the Key Idea

» Congratulate your learner & finish

General Notes: If your learner struggles with completing the worksheet, it is a clue that your student is focused on his/her own interests and hasn't been paying attention to friends.

That's okay. Communicate to your learner that being a friend means knowing what your friend is interested in.

Start with using a family member as the model for filling in the worksheet, as that should be easier. If you are adapting the task, make sure to stick with real people and not use characters from favorite TV shows or made-up characters that the student might like to talk about.

The next time you sit down to do social skills, stay with this worksheet. Work with your learner to role-play how they might find out this information from a friend. Their goal is to gather a little bit of information per day until they can fill in the chart for one or more friends.

Once your child can complete the worksheet for one or more friends, you are ready to move on.

Extra Practice: Choose additional friends and family members and talk about what you know about them. Ideally your learner can do this with little to no visual support.

After Session: As you encounter familiar people in daily life, ask your learner about things they know about that person. You can extend your learner's skill by getting them to come up with a question they could ask to learn more about their friend.

Your Notes/Extra Ideas:

2.1 Think About What I Know

When deciding what to talk to my friend about...

I think about what I know about my friend.

Choose two friends and fill in the information.

Likes		Recent Activities

Family News		Plans

Likes		Recent Activities

Family News		Plans

Coaching Guide: Choose A Shared Interest

Quick Reference:

> » Review the last worksheet
>
> » Introduce the Key Idea: Read, paraphrase, connect
>
> » Complete & review the worksheet
>
> » Extra practice
>
> » Revisit the Key Idea
>
> » Congratulate your learner & finish

General Notes: In this lesson, your learner starts making the connection between what they know about a person and how that affects what they ask and talk about with that person.

Make sure your learner uses a variety of questions rather than relying on a 'stock' question that gets them through many situations. You need your learner to practice the process of thinking about a person in order to choose an appropriate question.

Extra Practice: Go through different family members and friends and get your learner to identify two or three questions they could use to start a conversation. Your learner will need to think about interests, identify a shared interest and create a question. Great practice!

After Session: Prime your learner before social situations to think about some good questions to ask their friends/family members.

Your Notes/Extra Ideas:

2.2 Choose a Shared Interest

When deciding what to talk to my friend about...

I choose something my friend is interested in.

Draw a line from each topic to the friend that it suits best.

Likes
Minecraft
Soccer

Family News
New baby sister

Recent Activities
Went hiking
Studied math

Plans
Save for new phone
Go skiing

Likes
Cooking
Baseball

Family News
Dad got new job

Recent Activities
Baseball final
School field trip

Plans
Buy Pokemon cards

Who won baseball?

How is your sister doing?

How was hiking?

When are you getting
your Pokemon cards?

Have you decided which phone
you will buy?

Does your dad like his new job?

Now, look at the previous worksheet (2.1). For each friend write two questions you could ask to start a conversation with that friend.

------------------------------   ------------------------------

------------------------------   ------------------------------

Coaching Guide: Ask About Something Recent

Quick Reference:

> » Review the last worksheet
>
> » Introduce the Key Idea: Read, paraphrase, connect
>
> » Complete & review the worksheet
>
> » Extra practice
>
> » Revisit the Key Idea
>
> » Congratulate your learner & finish

General Notes: Even though your learner may be making great choices about topics, you may find they focus on aspects of the topic that are confusing to their friend. In the next three lessons, we provide guidelines for making better topic choices.

In this lesson, your learner practices asking about recent activities instead of ones from the past.

Extra Practice: Make up 3 or 4 more examples for your student to practice without visual support.

After Session: If necessary, provide gentle reminders for your learner in everyday situations.

Your Notes/Extra Ideas:

2.3 Ask About Something Recent

When deciding what to talk to my friend about...

I ask about something recent.

For each friend, choose the best question.

Did you go to Disneyland on the weekend?

Did you go to Disneyland three years ago?

Where did you have your birthday party when you were five?

Did you have a party for your birthday?

What did you have for dinner last night?

What did you have for dinner last week?

Coaching Guide: Ask For New Information

Quick Reference:

> » Review the last worksheet

> » Introduce the Key Idea: Read, Paraphrase, Connect

> » Complete & review the worksheet

> » Extra practice

> » Revisit the Key Idea

> » Congratulate your learner & finish

General Notes: ASD learners will often reuse a question that has been successful before. That is great, but friends can get tired of answering the same question, especially if the answer does not change from asking to asking.

Your learner needs to know that when we are making conversation, we should remember what we have asked before and ask something different this time.

Remind your learner that it is okay to re-ask the question if they actually need the information and have forgotten it.

Extra Practice: Make up 3 or 4 more examples for your student to practice without visual support.

After Session: If your learner asks you the same question too frequently, remind them to ask for new information.

Your Notes/Extra Ideas:

2.4 Ask For New Information

When deciding what to talk to my friend about...

I don't ask for information that he has told me before.

Which question is a better choice?

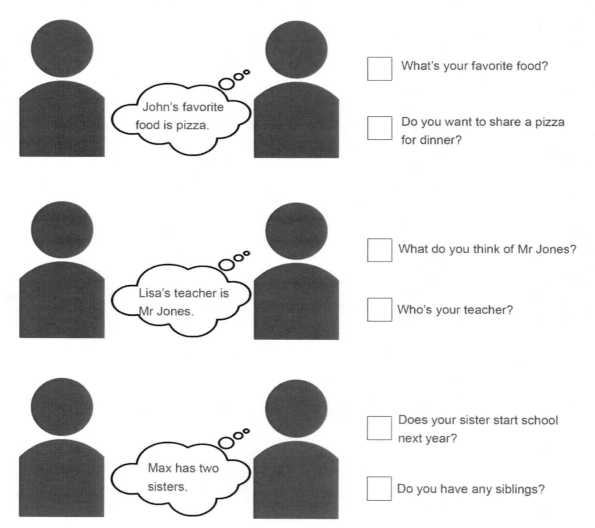

Coaching Guide: Remember Previous Conversations

Quick Reference:

» Review the last worksheet

» Introduce the Key Idea: Read, paraphrase, connect

» Complete & review the worksheet

» Extra practice

» Revisit the Key Idea

» Congratulate your learner & finish

General Notes: In this lesson, your learner practices using information he has heard to ask a relevant question that shows interest in his friend. This is a very important skill and may be quite challenging for your learner as it requires them to remember details from a previous conversation.

Students will get more practice at asking questions in the later chapter on follow-up questions. The key aspect of this worksheet is so that students know that they should remember information about their friends to use in later conversations.

Extra Practice: Make up 3 or 4 more examples for your student to practice without visual support. Use examples from the student's own life, or select from the following examples.

- Your friend Mila goes swimming every week. You think she may have a competition coming up soon. What is a good question to ask?

- Your uncle George competes in a pie baking contest every August. It is now September. What is a good question to ask?

- Your mom had an important meeting at work today. She has just come in the door. What is a good question to ask?

- Your dad plays tennis every Saturday. Today he is playing with a new partner. He arrives home after the game. What is a good question to ask?

After Session: Prime your learner before and after real-life conversations. After a conversation, get your learner to think about a good question for next time that shows that he was listening. Before a conversation, ask your learner to think of an interesting, relevant question.

2.5 Remember Previous Conversations

When deciding what to talk to my friend about...

I show that I remember what my friend has told me before.

Write a response that shows you remember what your friend said:

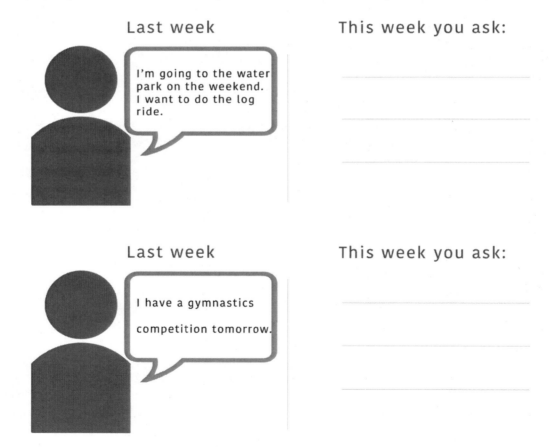

Last week

I'm going to the water park on the weekend. I want to do the log ride.

This week you ask:

_____

_____

_____

Last week

I have a gymnastics competition tomorrow.

This week you ask:

_____

_____

_____

Coaching Guide: Listen for Clues

Quick Reference:

> » Review the last worksheet
>
> » Introduce the Key Idea: Read, paraphrase, connect
>
> » Complete & review the worksheet
>
> » Extra practice
>
> » Revisit the Key Idea
>
> » Congratulate your learner & finish

General Notes: When a friend starts talking, their choice of topic tells us what they are interested in. In this lesson your learner practices identifying and attending to topics that their friend has introduced.

With this skill, your learner should reduce the amount he 'overrides' a peer's topic.

Extra Practice: Come up with additional examples, from real life if possible.

After Session: Prompt your learner to notice what topics his friends are interested in.

Your Notes/Extra Ideas:

2.6 Listen for Clues

When deciding what to talk to my friend about...

I should listen to the clues my friend gives me.

What does the speaker want to talk about?

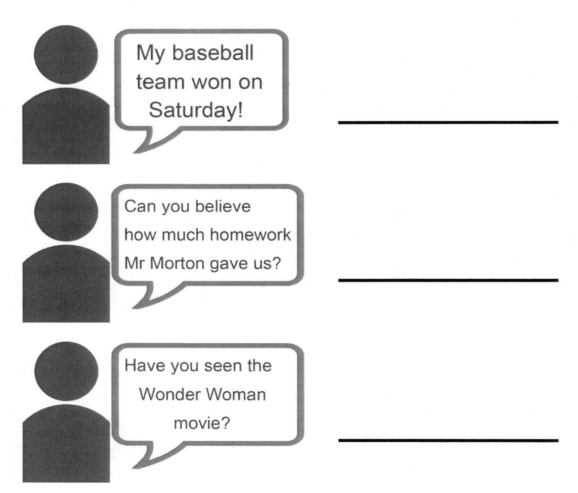

My baseball team won on Saturday!

_____

Can you believe how much homework Mr Morton gave us?

_____

Have you seen the Wonder Woman movie?

_____

Coaching Guide: Follow My Friend's Clues

Quick Reference:

> » Review the last worksheet
>
> » Introduce the Key Idea: Read, paraphrase, connect
>
> » Complete & review the worksheet
>
> » Extra practice
>
> » Revisit the Key Idea
>
> » Congratulate your learner & finish

General Notes: In this lesson your learner practices continuing on a friend's topic, rather than imposing his own topic.

You may need to spend time explaining how to read between the lines to figure out what a friend wants to talk about. The first example on the worksheet gives practice as your learner has to determine that the topic is not just about people getting mad, but about how the speaker feels about his mom.

Extra Practice: Come up with additional examples, ideally from real-life.

After Session: Prompt when your learner misses the clues in everyday situations.

Your Notes/Extra Ideas:

2.7 Follow My Friend's Clues

When deciding what to talk to my friend about...
I should follow my friend's clues and talk about what he wants to talk about.

Which response follows the clues given by the speaker?

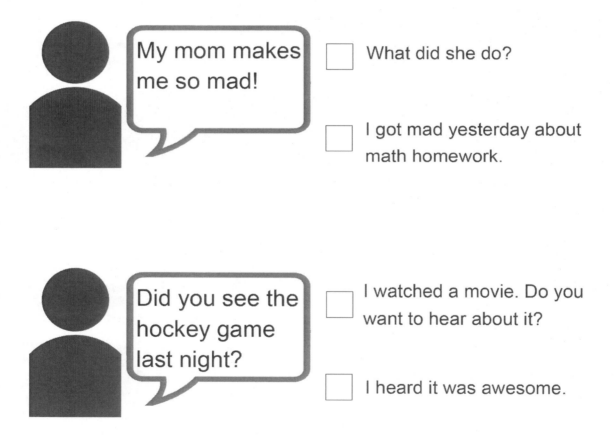

My mom makes me so mad!

☐ What did she do?

☐ I got mad yesterday about math homework.

Did you see the hockey game last night?

☐ I watched a movie. Do you want to hear about it?

☐ I heard it was awesome.

Coaching Guide: Check For Current Topic

Quick Reference:

> » Review the last worksheet

> » Introduce the Key Idea: Read, paraphrase, connect

> » Complete & review the worksheet

> » Extra practice

> » Revisit the Key Idea

> » Congratulate your learner & finish

General Notes: In this lesson, your learner practices paying attention to see if there is a topic that is already being talked about.

Kids with ASD tend to be focused on their own topics and often 'barge in' to a conversation. Learning to check first is a valuable skill.

After Session: Where possible, before your learner joins a group prime him/her to check if there is a current topic.

Your Notes/Extra Ideas:

2.8 Check for Current Topic

When deciding what to talk to my friend about...

I should check if there is already a topic being talked about.

What topic is already being talked about?

Did you see John's new phone?

Yeah. It's a super expensive model.

_____

Jax is moving to New York.

No way! When?

_____

Have you finished your art project?

Most of it. You?

_____

Coaching Guide: Choosing A Topic: Review

Quick Reference:

» Review the last worksheet

» Introduce the Key Idea: Read, paraphrase, connect

» Complete & review the worksheet

» Extra practice

» Revisit the Key Idea

» Congratulate your learner & finish

General Notes: Your learner has covered a lot of skills in this chapter. Use today as an opportunity to review those skills. Feel free to go back and review each of the worksheets individually.

It's okay if you take several sessions for review.

Extra Practice: Choose additional friends and identify good topics.

After Session: Continue to prompt/prime as needed, with the goal of fading the prompts as soon as possible.

Your Notes/Extra Ideas:

2.9 Choosing a Topic: Review

When deciding what to talk to my friend about...

I choose something they are interested in.

I choose something recent.

I show that I remember what my friend has already told me.

I listen for clues from my friend.

I check for topics already being talked about.

Think about 2 friends and come up with a good topic to talk to them about. Explain why it is a good topic.

WHO:_____

WHAT TOPIC:_____

WHY: _____

WHO:_____

WHAT TOPIC:_____

WHY: _____

Topic 3
Show I Am Listening

Background

An important part of continuing a conversation is to show we are listening. If we don't show we are listening, it looks like we are bored or not listening. In this case, the talker may disconnect from the conversation. That is not good for building a friendship!

In this section, students learn how to make short comments and actions that show they are listening and empathize with the talker.

Coaching Guide: Add a Short Comment

Quick Reference:

> » Review the last worksheet
>
> » Introduce the Key Idea: Read, paraphrase, connect
>
> » Complete & review the worksheet
>
> » Extra practice
>
> » Revisit the Key Idea
>
> » Congratulate your learner & finish

General Notes: Encourage your learner to use a variety of responses instead of just the same response every time. We focus on this issue in a later worksheet, but it is good to start off in the right way.

If your learner adds a follow-up question or comment (in addition to a short comment), that is fine. Focus any corrections just on the short comments as we will work on follow-up comments and follow-up questions later in this workbook.

Extra Practice: Tell your learner what happened in your day, or what your plans are, and require your learner to add short comments.

After Session: In everyday life, encourage your learner to show they are listening by adding a short comment.

Your Notes/Extra Ideas:

3.1 Add a Short Comment

When my friend does something or says something,
I can make a short comment like "Cool" or "Too bad."

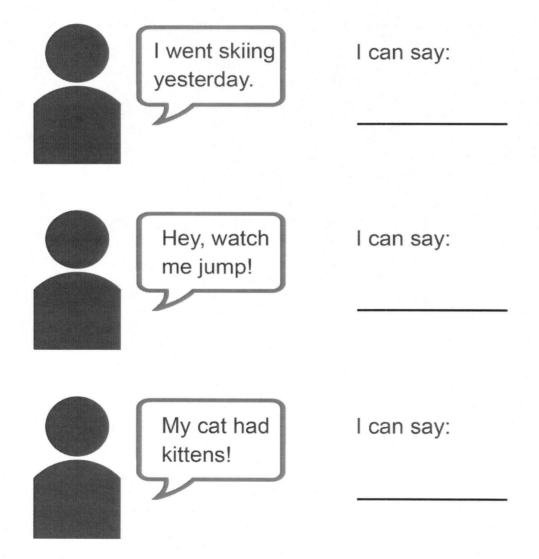

Coaching Guide: Match the Emotion

Quick Reference:

> » Review the last worksheet
>
> » Introduce the Key Idea: Read, paraphrase, connect
>
> » Complete & review the worksheet
>
> » Extra practice
>
> » Revisit the Key Idea
>
> » Congratulate your learner & finish

General Notes: In this lesson your student learns to attend to the emotion of his friend and match his comment to that emotion.

Extra Practice: Make a variety of statements that range from happy to sad, fun to boring, and help your learner notice the emotion and make an appropriate response.

After Session: Encourage your learner to make appropriate responses to his family and peers.

Your Notes/Extra Ideas:

3.2 Match the Emotion

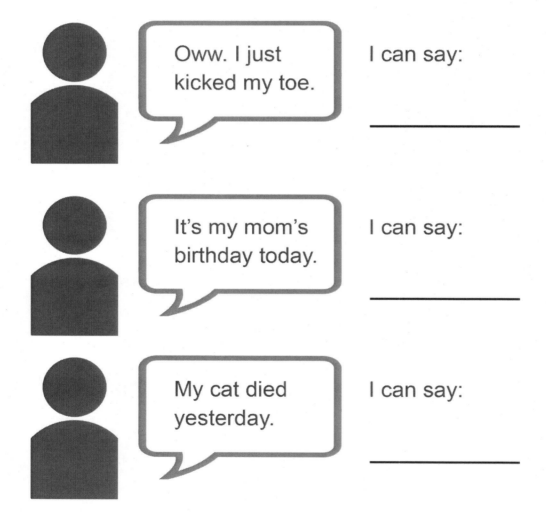

Oww. I just kicked my toe.

I can say:

_____

It's my mom's birthday today.

I can say:

_____

My cat died yesterday.

I can say:

_____

Coaching Guide: Vary What I Say

Quick Reference:

> » Review the last worksheet
>
> » Introduce the Key Idea: Read, paraphrase, connect
>
> » Complete & review the worksheet
>
> » Extra practice
>
> » Revisit the Key Idea
>
> » Congratulate your learner & finish

General Notes: Encourage your learner to use a wide variety of responses. Sometimes ASD learners want to simplify their responses to something like "Cool" and "That's too bad." Right from the beginning you need to encourage variety.

Extra Practice: Make a variety of comments that range from happy to sad, fun to boring, and help your learner notice the emotion and make appropriate varying responses.

After Session: Encourage your learner to make varied responses to his family and peers.

Your Notes/Extra Ideas:

3.3 Vary What I Say

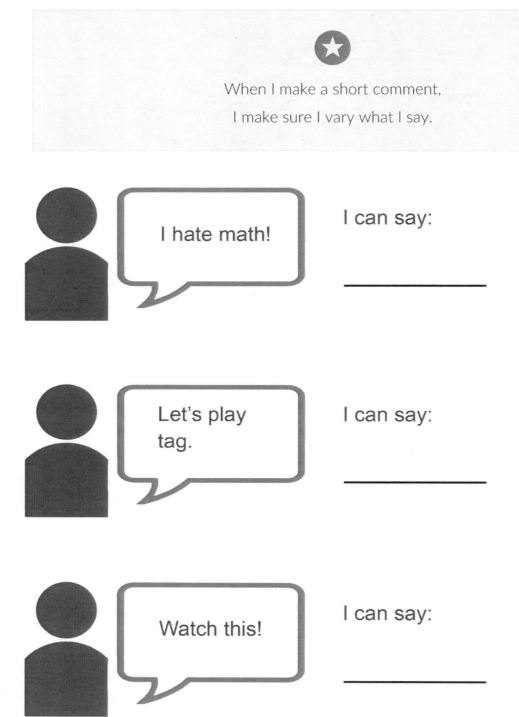

I hate math!　　　I can say:

_____

Let's play tag.　　　I can say:

_____

Watch this!　　　I can say:

_____

Coaching Guide: Use Eyes and Body

Quick Reference:

> » Review the last worksheet

> » Introduce the Key Idea: Read, paraphrase, connect

> » Complete & review the worksheet

> » Extra practice

> » Revisit the Key Idea

> » Congratulate your learner & finish

General Notes: Firstly, please note that some Autistic individuals find eye contact extremely aversive. Do not force your learner to make eye contact.

Your goal is to help your learner understand WHY looking towards our conversation partner can be useful. If they are comfortable with it, help them practice.

In this lesson, we talk about gaze direction because looking toward our partner is an easy way to communicate that we are listening. Smiles, nods and other gestures can also be used to show you are attending to your friend.

Encourage your child to try all of these in this safe practice situation with you. Help them figure out what non-verbal communication strategies work best for them.

Extra Practice: Spend a few minutes where your learner can ONLY show they are listening with their eyes and/or body.

After Session: Encourage your learner to show they are listening using their eyes, body or a short comment.

Your Notes/Extra Ideas:

3.4 Use Eyes and Body

If my friend is looking at me, I can show I am listening with my eyes and my body. The important thing is to show that I heard.

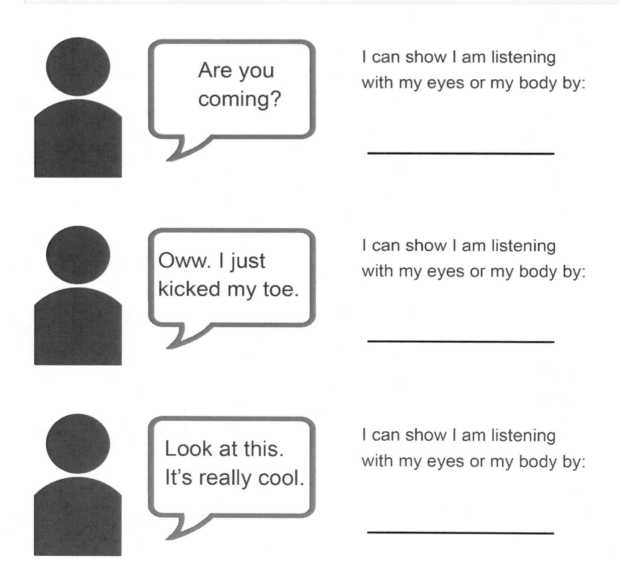

Are you coming?

I can show I am listening with my eyes or my body by:

_____

Oww. I just kicked my toe.

I can show I am listening with my eyes or my body by:

_____

Look at this. It's really cool.

I can show I am listening with my eyes or my body by:

_____

Coaching Guide: Let's Practice

Quick Reference:

- » Review the last worksheet

- » Introduce the Key Idea: Read, paraphrase, connect

- » Complete & review the worksheet

- » Extra practice

- » Revisit the Key Idea

- » Congratulate your learner & finish

General Notes: Instead of filling in the worksheet, a great way to practice is for the coach to make the statement and for the learner to respond to the coach. This is much more like real conversation and will help with generalization of the skills.

Extra Practice: Keep making comments for your learner to respond to.

After Session: Increase your expectations about how your learner will respond to family and friends in real life. Prompt as needed until prompts can be faded.

Your Notes/Extra Ideas:

3.5 Let's Practice

Let's practice showing we are listening.

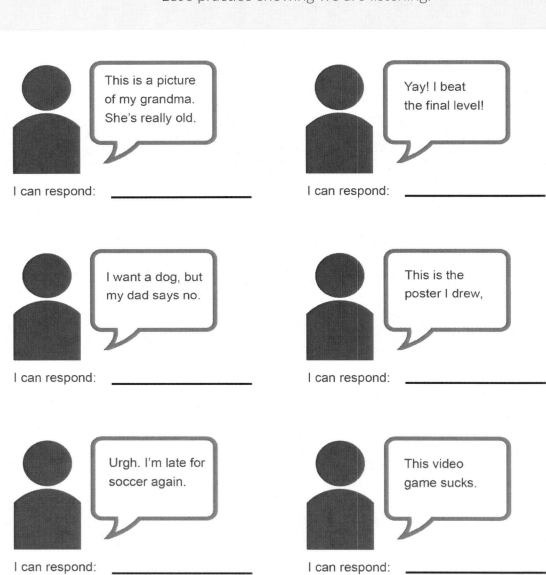

This is a picture of my grandma. She's really old.

I can respond: _____

Yay! I beat the final level!

I can respond: _____

I want a dog, but my dad says no.

I can respond: _____

This is the poster I drew,

I can respond: _____

Urgh. I'm late for soccer again.

I can respond: _____

This video game sucks.

I can respond: _____

Coaching Guide: Review

Quick Reference:

» Review the last worksheet

» Introduce the Key Idea: Read, paraphrase, connect

» Complete & review the worksheet

» Extra practice

» Revisit the Key Idea

» Congratulate your learner & finish

General Notes: Today consists of more practice. It can be handy to note down a few of your learner's responses so that your learner can check them against the checklist at the bottom of the page.

Your Notes/Extra Ideas:

3.6 Review

Review.

Practice with your coach.

My coach said: _____

I responded with: _____

My coach said: _____

I responded with: _____

My coach said: _____

I responded with: _____

My coach said: _____

I responded with: _____

CHECKLIST

☐ I used my body to show I was listening   ☐ I varied my words

☐ I matched the speaker's emotion

Topic 4
Ask a Follow-up Question

Background

In this section, your student learns how to ask an appropriate, on-topic follow-up question when their friend has said something. A follow-up question is a question that is related to the current topic of conversation.

Some examples of appropriate follow-up questions are:

A: I went to Playland yesterday!

B: That sounds like fun! What rides did you go on?

A: We went camping on the weekend.

B: Cool. Where did you go?

Follow-up questions are often preceded by a short comment, as illustrated in the previous examples.

Coaching Guide: Ask a Follow-up Question

Quick Reference:

> » Review the last worksheet

> » Introduce the Key Idea: Read, paraphrase, connect

> » Complete & review the worksheet

> » Extra practice

> » Revisit the Key Idea

> » Congratulate your learner & finish

General Notes: Encourage your learner to identify more than one follow-up question per statement. Usually there are many possible follow-up questions and it is good for your learner to know this.

Extra Practice: Make statements about what happened recently and require some follow-up questions from your learner.

After Session: Encourage follow-up questions during conversations.

Your Notes/Extra Ideas:

4.1 Ask a Follow-up Question

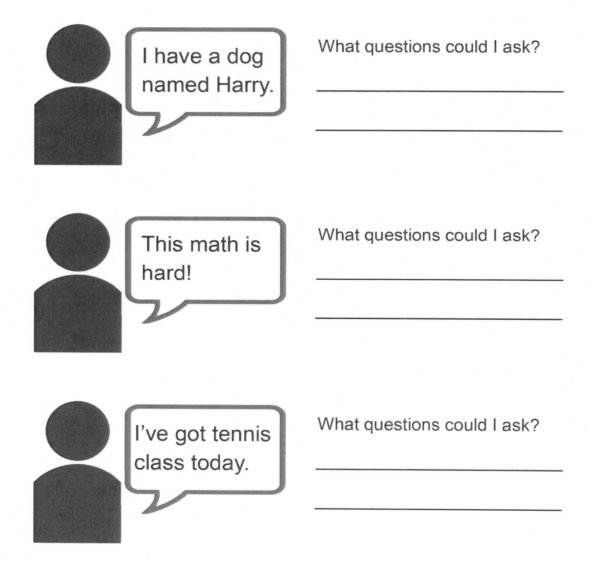

I have a dog named Harry.

What questions could I ask?

_____

_____

This math is hard!

What questions could I ask?

_____

_____

I've got tennis class today.

What questions could I ask?

_____

_____

Coaching Guide: Make it Related

Quick Reference:

> » Review the last worksheet
>
> » Introduce the Key Idea: Read, paraphrase, connect
>
> » Complete & review the worksheet
>
> » Extra practice
>
> » Revisit the Key Idea
>
> » Congratulate your learner & finish

General Notes: Children with ASD often struggle with following the intent of a friend's statement so they may have trouble making their follow-up questions 'on topic.' Help your learner think about WHY his friend made the statement. That will help your learner ask a relevant follow-up question.

For example, when a friend tells you he got a new video game he is probably excited about the game. He probably wants you to ask about the game.

Extra Practice: Provide more examples for your student to practice with.

After Session: Encourage on-topic follow-up questions in everyday life.

Your Notes/Extra Ideas:

4.2 Make It Related

My follow-up question must be **related** to what my friend said. This is called being 'on topic.'

My dad bought a new car.

Which question is related?

☐ What type of car did he buy?

☐ I saw a strange car yesterday.

It's going to snow tonight.

Which question is related?

☐ Do you have math homework?

☐ Did they say how much snow?

I got the new Mario game.

Which question is related?

☐ Which one?

☐ Do you play chess?

Coaching Guide: Ask for New Information

Quick Reference:

>> Review the last worksheet

>> Introduce the Key Idea: Read, paraphrase, connect

>> Complete & review the worksheet

>> Extra practice

>> Revisit the Key Idea

>> Congratulate your learner & finish

General Notes: Sometimes children with ASD ask for information that you KNOW that they already know. This worksheet helps learners think about what they already know and ask about what they don't yet know.

Your Notes/Extra Ideas:

4.3 Ask for New Information

My follow-up question should not ask for information I know already. I ask for **new** information.

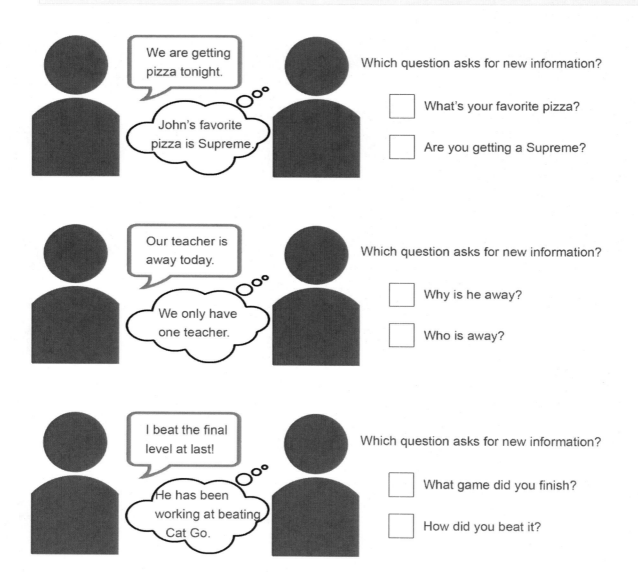

We are getting pizza tonight.

John's favorite pizza is Supreme.

Which question asks for new information?

☐ What's your favorite pizza?

☐ Are you getting a Supreme?

Our teacher is away today.

We only have one teacher.

Which question asks for new information?

☐ Why is he away?

☐ Who is away?

I beat the final level at last!

He has been working at beating Cat Go.

Which question asks for new information?

☐ What game did you finish?

☐ How did you beat it?

Coaching Guide: *Keep to My Friend's Topic*

Quick Reference:

» Review the last worksheet

» Introduce the Key Idea: Read, paraphrase, connect

» Complete & review the worksheet

» Extra practice

» Revisit the Key Idea

» Congratulate your learner & finish

General Notes: Many children with ASD have special interests that they spend a lot of time thinking about and talking about. When asking a follow-up question, they may connect the topic to their own special interest.

Use this worksheet to help your learner consider what their friend said and think about what their friend probably wants to talk about.

After Session: In everyday life, help your learner think about what their friends want to talk about.

Your Notes/Extra Ideas:

4.4 Keep to My Friend's Topic

My follow-up question should be related to my friend's interests, not my own special interests.

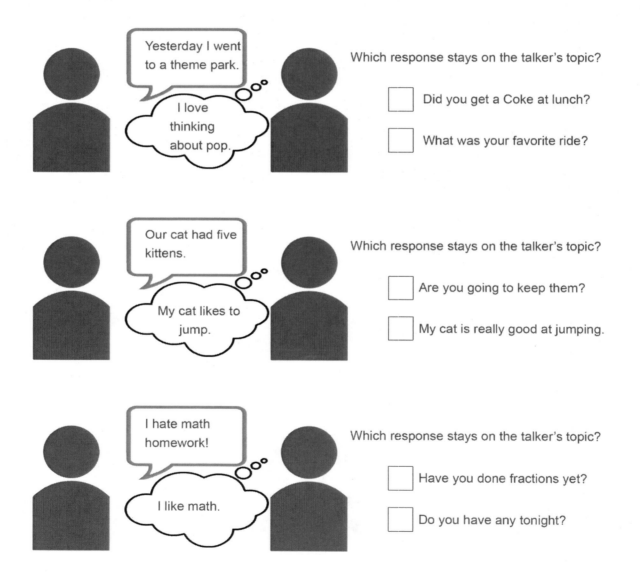

Coaching Guide: Use Open Questions

Quick Reference:

> » Review the last worksheet
>
> » Introduce the Key Idea: Read, paraphrase, connect
>
> » Complete & review the worksheet
>
> » Extra practice
>
> » Revisit the Key Idea
>
> » Congratulate your learner & finish

General Notes: Open questions are 'what', 'when', 'where', etc, questions which allow for a more informative answer. They differ from Yes/No questions which can only be answered with a Yes or a No.

Open questions show that you want to know more about the topic. For example,

A: What did you do at the theme park?

B: I went on all the roller coasters five times!

Yes/No questions don't allow for the responder to add much information.

A: Did you go on the Ferris wheel?

B: No

Too many Yes/No questions can also sound like an interrogation.

A: Did you go on the Ferris wheel?

B: No.

A: Did you go on the carousel?

B: No.

A: Did you eat lunch at McDonalds?

B: No.

With today's worksheet, you help your learner use WH questions. If your learner has previously been an 'interrogator', you'll be surprised at how much easier it is to have a conversation.

After Session: Real-life might need quite a bit of prompting. It is worth it for the improvement in conversation skill.

4.5 Use Open Questions

Good follow-up questions are 'open' questions that start with WHEN, WHERE, WHY, WHO, HOW, WHAT, etc.

Think of some follow-up questions for these statements.

I went skating on the weekend.

When
_____
Where
_____
Who
_____
How
_____
Why
_____
What
_____

My dad got really mad at me yesterday.

When
_____
Where
_____
Who
_____
How
_____
Why
_____
What
_____

Coaching Guide: Let's Practice Open Questions

Quick Reference:

» Review the last worksheet

» Introduce the Key Idea: Read, paraphrase, connect

» Complete & review the worksheet

» Extra practice

» Revisit the Key Idea

» Congratulate your learner & finish

General Notes: We include a second day of practice for WH questions. You can use this time to also consolidate the skill of asking for **new** information that is **related** to the friend's interests.

Your Notes/Extra Ideas:

4.6 Let's Practice Open Questions

Let's practice more 'open' follow-up questions.

Think of some follow-up questions for these statements.

My teacher crashed his car on the way to school.

When
_____

Where
_____

Who
_____

How
_____

Why
_____

What
_____

I really want to get some more Pokémon cards.

When
_____

Where
_____

Who
_____

How
_____

Why
_____

What
_____

Coaching Guide: Look When I Start Talking

Quick Reference:

> » Review the last worksheet

> » Introduce the Key Idea: Read, paraphrase, connect

> » Complete & review the worksheet

> » Extra practice

> » Revisit the Key Idea

> » Congratulate your learner & finish

General Notes: Today's focus is another lesson about how neurotypical individuals use gaze direction (where we look) and body language to communicate.

In this lesson, your learner will practice using gaze direction and/or body language to communicate who they are directing their question to.

If eye contact is aversive for your learner, help them figure out a strategy that works for them. Perhaps turning their mouth or body towards their listener will feel more comfortable.

The goal is effective communication – not uncomfortable communication - so let your learner determine what is best for them.

After Session: Like many of the skills in this book, practice during everyday life is needed to really cement the skill.

Your Notes/Extra Ideas:

4.7 Look When I Start Talking

I can look toward my friend briefly when I ask my follow-up question so that he knows I am talking to him.

Practice follow-up questions with your coach. He or she will score every follow-up question.

Looked toward Me During Follow-up Question	Did Not Look toward Me During Follow-up Question

Save this score sheet for later. Do it again in a week or two. Did you score better?

Looked toward Me During Follow-up Question	Did Not Look toward Me During Follow-up Question

Coaching Guide: Review

Quick Reference:

> » Review the last worksheet
>
> » Introduce the Key Idea: Read, paraphrase, connect
>
> » Complete & review the worksheet
>
> » Extra practice
>
> » Revisit the Key Idea
>
> » Congratulate your learner & finish

General Notes: Today is a chance to practice bringing all the skills together. Have fun with scoring each other.

Your Notes/Extra Ideas:

4.8 Review

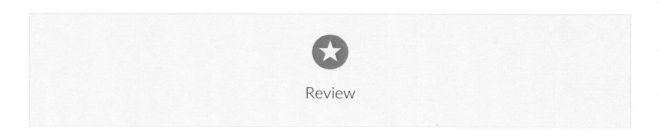

Review

Practice making follow-up questions with your coach.

You can use the following checklist to score each other.

☐ On topic

☐ Asked for new information

☐ Is related to my friend's interests

☐ Is an open question using a WH word

☐ Included body language/gaze direction comfortably and appropriately

Topic 5
Add a Follow-up Comment

Background

In this section, students learn to make follow-up comments. A follow-up comment is a comment where the speaker adds some information relevant to what was just said.

For example:

      A: I went to the movies on the weekend.

      B: Hey, so did I!

In this conversation the 'so did I' is a follow-up comment. It is relevant additional information to the topic that speaker A introduced.

Follow-up comments are typically used as an alternative to follow-up questions.

Coaching Guide: Add a Follow-up Comment

Quick Reference:

> » Review the last worksheet
>
> » Introduce the Key Idea: Read, paraphrase, connect
>
> » Complete & review the worksheet
>
> » Extra practice
>
> » Revisit the Key Idea
>
> » Congratulate your learner & finish

General Notes: At first, your student may have trouble switching from follow-up questions to follow-up comments. Think of a follow-up comment as adding new information to the current topic.

After Session: Encourage follow-up comments in everyday life.

5.1 Add a Follow-up Comment

After my friend says something, I can make a short comment and add a **follow-up comment**.

This means I add information to what my friend said.

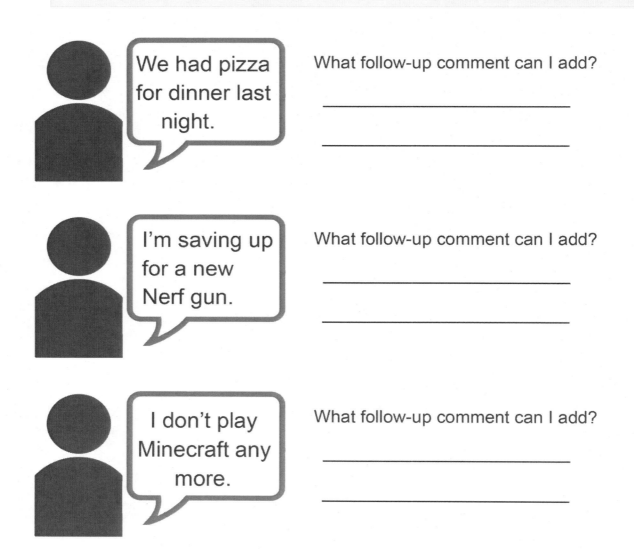

We had pizza for dinner last night.

What follow-up comment can I add?

_____

_____

I'm saving up for a new Nerf gun.

What follow-up comment can I add?

_____

_____

I don't play Minecraft any more.

What follow-up comment can I add?

_____

_____

Coaching Guide: Make It Related

Quick Reference:

> » Review the last worksheet
>
> » Introduce the Key Idea: Read, paraphrase, connect
>
> » Complete & review the worksheet
>
> » Extra practice
>
> » Revisit the Key Idea
>
> » Congratulate your learner & finish

General Notes: Your learner's follow-up comment must be related to the speaker's topic and intention. Watch out for your learner relating the speaker's topics to his own special interests. You may need to help your learner think about what his friend wants to talk about.

Your Notes/Extra Ideas:

5.2 Make It Related

My follow-up comment should be **related** to what my friend said. This is being 'on-topic.'

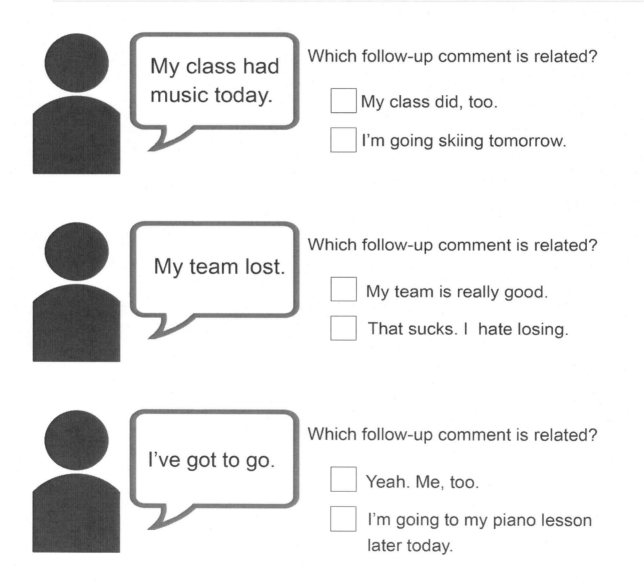

My class had music today.

Which follow-up comment is related?

☐ My class did, too.

☐ I'm going skiing tomorrow.

My team lost.

Which follow-up comment is related?

☐ My team is really good.

☐ That sucks. I hate losing.

I've got to go.

Which follow-up comment is related?

☐ Yeah. Me, too.

☐ I'm going to my piano lesson later today.

Coaching Guide: Give New Information

Quick Reference:

» Review the last worksheet

» Introduce the Key Idea: Read, paraphrase, connect

» Complete & review the worksheet

» Extra practice

» Revisit the Key Idea

» Congratulate your learner & finish

General Notes: Learners with ASD will often happily tell you information they have told you before. Help your learner realize that they should be giving information that is new to their listener. Listeners do not want to hear information they already know.

Extra Practice: If your learner struggles, provide extra practice.

Your Notes/Extra Ideas:

5.3 Give New Information

My follow-up comment should contain information that is **new** to my friend. This means he doesn't know that information already.

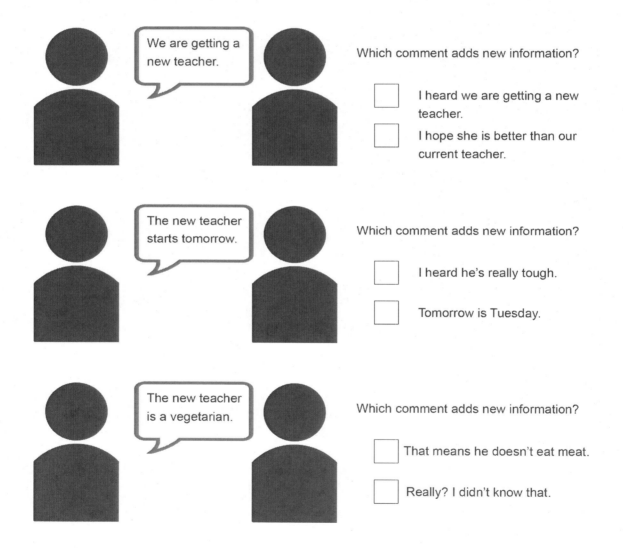

We are getting a new teacher.

Which comment adds new information?

☐ I heard we are getting a new teacher.

☐ I hope she is better than our current teacher.

The new teacher starts tomorrow.

Which comment adds new information?

☐ I heard he's really tough.

☐ Tomorrow is Tuesday.

The new teacher is a vegetarian.

Which comment adds new information?

☐ That means he doesn't eat meat.

☐ Really? I didn't know that.

Coaching Guide: Use Variety

Quick Reference:

> » Review the last worksheet
>
> » Introduce the Key Idea: Read, paraphrase, connect
>
> » Complete & review the worksheet
>
> » Extra practice
>
> » Revisit the Key Idea
>
> » Congratulate your learner & finish

General Notes: ASD learners can get rigid in how they respond. In this lesson, your student learns that it is okay to have variety in how he replies. He can do just a short comment, or a short comment and a follow-up comment, or just a follow-up comment.

Extra Practice: Keep making statements and encouraging variety in responses.

Your Notes/Extra Ideas:

5.4 Use Variety

I can do a **short comment** AND a **follow-up comment**. Or I can do just one of them.

My dad lost his job.

Respond to your friend.

_____

_____

My sister has a boyfriend.

Respond to your friend.

_____

_____

I'm going to soccer camp in the summer.

Respond to your friend.

_____

_____

Coaching Guide: Use My Eyes

Quick Reference:

> » Review the last worksheet
>
> » Introduce the Key Idea: Read, paraphrase, connect
>
> » Complete & review the worksheet
>
> » Extra practice
>
> » Revisit the Key Idea
>
> » Congratulate your learner & finish

General Notes: Yet again we touch on how gaze and general body language can be used to communicate.

Please remember that eye contact can be aversive to your learner. Your goal is to help them figure out a strategy for non-verbally communicating that they are addressing their conversation partner. Often, just turning their face towards the intended person is enough.

Extra Practice: Practice and review this lesson until your learner naturally uses gaze/body language to comfortably and appropriately communicate who they are talking to.

After Session: Raise your expectations with regards to this skill during everyday life.

Your Notes/Extra Ideas:

5.5 Use My Eyes

When I start a follow-up comment, I can look toward my friend so he knows I am talking to him.

Practice follow-up comments with your coach. He or she will score every follow-up comment.

Looked at Me During Follow-up Comment	Did Not Look at Me During Follow-up Comment

Save this score sheet for later. Do it again in a week or two. Did you score better?

Looked at Me During Follow-up Comment	Did Not Look at Me During Follow-up Comment

Coaching Guide: Review

Quick Reference:

> » Review the last worksheet
>
> » Introduce the Key Idea: Read, paraphrase, connect
>
> » Complete & review the worksheet
>
> » Extra practice
>
> » Revisit the Key Idea
>
> » Congratulate your learner & finish

General Notes: Today is a chance to practice all the skills together. Have fun with scoring each other.

Your Notes/Extra Ideas:

5.6 Review

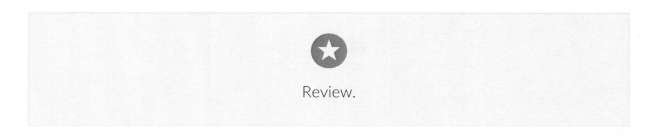

Review.

Practice making follow-up comments with your coach. You can add some follow-up questions as well if it feels natural.

You can use the following checklist to score each other.

☐ On topic

☐ Gave new information

☐ Is related to my friend's topic/interests

☐ Included body language/gaze direction comfortably and appropriately

Topic 6
Make Conversation

Background

In this section, students practice extended conversations by using a mix of short comments, follow-up questions and follow-up comments.

Your learner has come a long way!

Coaching Guide: Use Variety

Quick Reference:

» Review the last worksheet

» Introduce the Key Idea: Read, paraphrase, connect

» Complete & review the worksheet

» Extra practice

» Revisit the Key Idea

» Congratulate your learner & finish

General Notes: In this lesson make sure that your learner can fluently respond to conversational statements using both follow-up comments and follow-up questions. It is fine if your student appropriately uses both in a response.

If your learner struggles, remember that you can make one statement and get your learner to brainstorm multiple responses to that one statement.

Extra Practice: Keep talking ☺

Your Notes/Extra Ideas:

6.1 Use Variety

When my friend says something, I can use a follow-up question or a follow-up comment. It is good to mix it up.

Coach: Choose a topic and say something. Your learner should respond with a follow-up question or comment. Tally how often each is used to make sure there is variety.

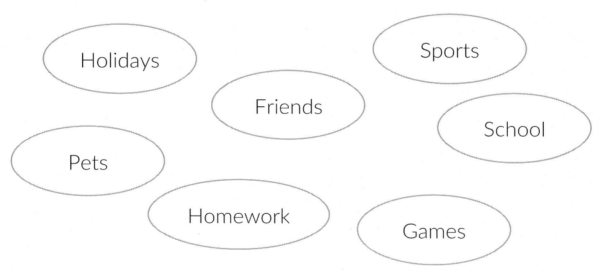

Follow-up Comments	Follow-up Questions

Coaching Guide: Let's Practice

Quick Reference:

> » Review the last worksheet
>
> » Introduce the Key Idea: Read, paraphrase, connect
>
> » Complete & review the worksheet
>
> » Extra practice
>
> » Revisit the Key Idea
>
> » Congratulate your learner & finish

General Notes: Today's lesson involves more practice at responding fluently with follow-up questions and follow-up comments.

Your Notes/Extra Ideas:

6.2 Let's Practice

Let's practice some more.

Coach: Choose a topic and say something. Your learner should respond with a follow-up question or comment. Tally how often each is used to make sure there is variety.

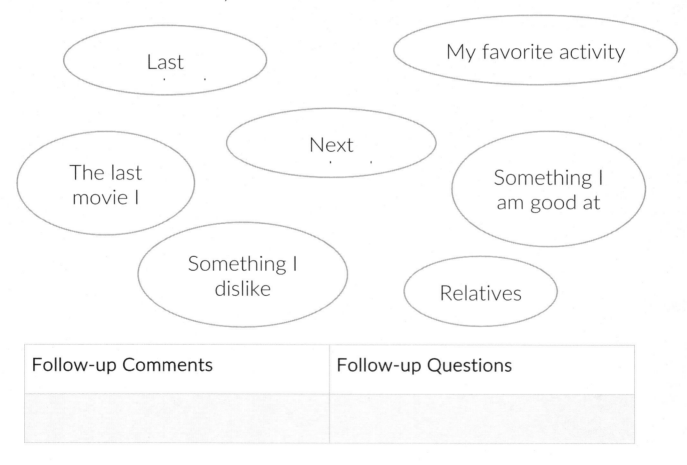

Follow-up Comments	Follow-up Questions

Coaching Guide: Two Turns Each

Quick Reference:

>> Review the last worksheet

>> Introduce the Key Idea: Read, paraphrase, connect

>> Complete & review the worksheet

>> Extra practice

>> Revisit the Key Idea

>> Congratulate your learner & finish

General Notes: Over the next few sessions, you focus on extending the number of turns that you talk back and forth. Keep all the Key Ideas in mind. Make sure your learner's responses are on-topic, new and varied.

Note weaknesses and spend a session or two reviewing that worksheet.

Your Notes/Extra Ideas:

6.3 Two Turns Each

Using follow-up comments and follow-up questions, my friend and I can keep

talking about a topic.

Goal: 2 turns each

Choose a topic and keep talking until you have had two turns each. Use these topics or choose your own.

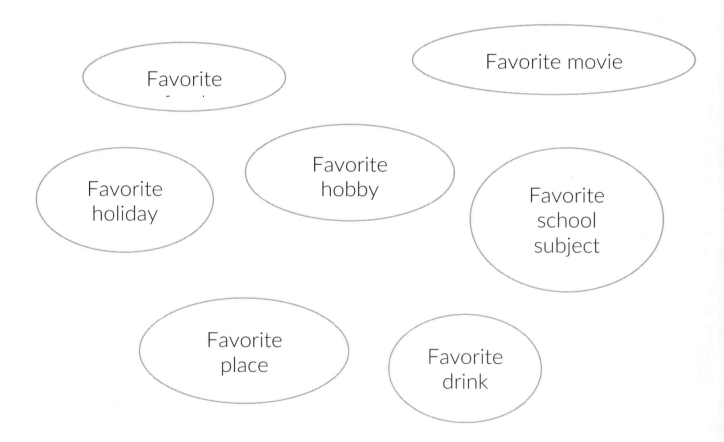

Coaching Guide: Three Turns Each

Quick Reference:

> » Review the last worksheet
>
> » Introduce the Key Idea: Read, paraphrase, connect
>
> » Complete & review the worksheet
>
> » Extra practice
>
> » Revisit the Key Idea
>
> » Congratulate your learner & finish

General Notes: Your conversations should extend to three turns each. Don't feel like you need to rigidly stay on the same topic. It is okay for the topic to gradually morph – as long as it is a natural progression that meets all the key ideas.

Your Notes/Extra Ideas:

6.4 Three Turns Each

Using follow-up comments and follow-up questions, my friend and I can keep talking about a topic.

Goal: 3 turns each

Choose a topic and keep talking until you have had three turns each. Use these topics or choose your own.

What do you want for your

What musical instrument would you like to play?

What is your least favorite subject?

What do you want to be when you grow up?

What book do you love the most?

Where do you want to live when you grow up?

Coaching Guide: Four Turns Each

Quick Reference:

» Review the last worksheet

» Introduce the Key Idea: Read, paraphrase, connect

» Complete & review the worksheet

» Extra practice

» Revisit the Key Idea

» Congratulate your learner & finish

General Notes: Your conversation should extend to four turns each. As mentioned previously, the topic of conversation can change, as long as the Key Idea criteria are met.

Your Notes/Extra Ideas:

6.5 Four Turns Each

Using follow-up comments and follow-up questions, my friend and I can keep talking about a topic.

Goal: 4 turns each

Choose a topic and keep talking until you have had four turns each. Use these topics or choose your own.

What was fun this

Would you rather be youngest or oldest?

What video game world would you like to live in?

What is your favorite thing to do as a family?

What is your favorite thing to do by yourself?

What would you do if you were the

Coaching Guide: Review

Quick Reference:

 » Review the last worksheet

 » Introduce the Key Idea: Read, paraphrase, connect

 » Complete & review the worksheet

 » Extra practice

 » Revisit the Key Idea

 » Congratulate your learner & finish

General Notes: The final day of practice. Use the checklist on each other as a final check of proficiency. Celebrate the progress with your learner!

Your Notes/Extra Ideas:

6.6 Review

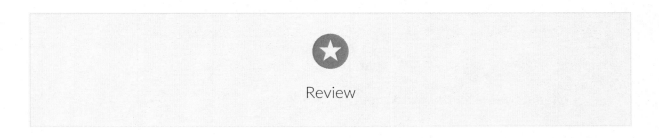

Review

Today's goal is to just talk! Coach, use the following checklist to identify any areas that need a bit more review.

Checklist:

☐ On topic

☐ Gives new information

☐ Is related to my friend's topic/interests

☐ Includes appropriate and comfortable body language/gaze.

☐ Includes both comments and questions in the conversation

CERTIFICATE OF ACHIEVEMENT

THIS CERTIFICATE IS AWARDED TO

_____

IN RECOGNITION OF

_____

_____   _____

DATE   SIGNATURE

What Next?

Look out for the next in our Six-Minute Social Skills series!

Available on Amazon or at www.HappyFrogPress.com

Key Ideas Summary

Download a one-page summary of all the Key Ideas introduced in the workbook.

Great for quick reference!

Available for free on our website:

HappyFrogLearning.com/product/Conversation_Key_Ideas

Need More Resources?

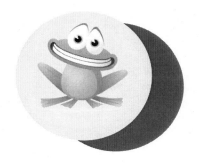

www.HappyFrogLearning.com

Happy Frog Learning creates quality resources for elementary-aged and high school children with autism and other social/language challenges.

Our award-winning apps, workbooks and curriculums target reading comprehension, social skills and writing.

Visit our website today to learn more.

Made in United States
North Haven, CT
24 February 2024

49141667R00063